A Way To Stop Smoking
Before Its Too Late

Other books by this author

The Number One Secret To
Permanent Weight Loss

All books available now on
Amazon.com

A Way To Stop Smoking
Before Its Too Late

2009

How I quit smoking 15 years ago and you can too!

Table Of Contents

Chapter One

Do You Really One To Quit Smoking?

Well the first question you need to be asking yourself right now and serious contemplating it are you really ready to give them up. This is the most important step in quitting is this very question because any method of smoking cessation that you try is going to end up in another failed attempt if you don't first really and truly make up your mind that you are indeed ready to do this.

You and your desire to quit smoking are truly the first and most important step in not only quitting smoking but in anything you wish to try and accomplish in your life first must be approached with you and your personal responsibility for your actions, habits good or bad it is truly up to you to affect the positive change in your life that you seek.

One of the number one reasons people hesitate to start or try a smoking cessation plan is they believe and have heard from many people that say they will gain weight with stopping smoking. This is certainly something one must consider when thinking about quitting smoking. I know that I personally gained about 20 pounds myself when I stopped smoking but when I stopped to think about the risks of smoking versus the risks of being overweight there is not much in the comparison that would put me on the side of continuing to smoke. I would much rather take my chance on the problems associated with weight gain than I ever would with fighting cancer.

I watched helplessly as my own brother died of brain cancer. He suffered so severely in his death bed. It was hour after agonizing hour watching slowly die and holding his hand as he would struggle and gasp for each breath trying to get enough air into his lungs to survive. I had to listen to him over and over wheezing to get just the smallest amount of air into his dying body and listening to him plead with us to put him on a breathing machine and hearing him in the faintest whisper of all he could muster up to say "I can't breathe, I can't breathe with his eyes wide open with fear as he knew his life was slowly slipping away from him. I can remember going to the bathroom when I could not take any more and getting down on my knees on that cold tile floor and begging, crying out to God PLEASE LORD JUST TAKE HIM HOME WITH YOU RIGHT NOW AND DON'T LET HIM SUFFER ANYMORE! I would do this repeatedly throughout the night as he continued his slow death of suffocating second by second minute by minute hour by hour. It's not much fun watching someone you love die when there is not a thing in the world you can do to help them. We were told a breathing machine would not help him because of all the blood clotting that was in his lungs. Think long and hard about this kind of death the next time you light up.

There are simple things you can do as to avoid gaining weight when stop smoking. The biggest thing is not to replace one bad habit with another. Instead of grabbing a cigarette you start grabbing candy bars and that sort of thing and you will be doomed to putting on extra pounds but again I still say even if you gain some weight it is certainly a much lesser of two evils in my opinion.

There are still other ways you can prevent yourself from possibly gaining weight. You will be amazed at how much more energy you will have after stopping smoking and you can begin any number if different exercise programs that can even further benefit you health. You can go for a walk around the block on your 'smoke breaks' that you use to take can be turned into 'health breaks' and go for a walk.

Another obstacle you must be aware of is not everyone will be as excited about your stopping smoking. When I tried to quit the first few time I unfortunately worked with people who would like nothing better than to see me fail at stopping smoking and even did what they could to encourage me not to quit. They would say stuff like "Ah you ain't gonna quit." "Come on man here's you a cigarette!" and would basically push them in front of my face trying to get me to smoke one. Yeah that's a good friend you have when they are trying to do that and you can pretty much figure someone like that is not much of a friend or they would try to encourage you in your quest for better health instead trying to undermine your efforts. I am sad to report that their negative effort had their intended poisonous effect on me and many times I ended up back on cigarettes because of people like this so beware of this and know and mentally prepare that there may be someone you know who might try this one on you. This made it all that much harder for me when I finally did devise a plan to stop smoking once and for all.

Another challenge for you will be of course what to do with your hands! If you smoke a pack a day you are literally not only in the habit of the smoking but you are in the habit of hundreds of times a day putting your hand to your mouth to take a draw and then there is the endless playing with the cigarettes of the ritual flicking of ashes hundreds of time a day. You may do yourself a favor of keeping toothpicks to play with or a rubbing rock or just take a coin out of your pocket and fidget with it. The bottom line with any method of stopping smoking that you eventually try is never giving up. Keep trying and trying and trying and if you really really want to you will find a way to give them up. I cannot express to you how strongly you must want to quit before it will happen. And half-hearted attempt will be just that half quitting is not quitting you. Once you are sure your desire is there and your mind is set on quitting cigarettes then you are ready for what I believe is the easiest and least expensive way to stop.

This brings to me yet another topic and that is money! First of all the cigarette tobacco industry is a multi-billion dollar industry so don't the few lawsuits they don't win is going to put them out of business any time soon and my oh my just think of all the wasted money that is spent on your habit by you. If you smoke a pack a day at $5.oo a pack and that's rough average, I know they are a little more and a little less in different places but for sake of the example let's just say five bucks a pack and you smoke a pack a day that comes to $1,825 a year! That's $35.oo dollars a week. I don't know about you but I get paid at my current "day" job every two weeks so if I still smoked a pack a day that a whopping $75.oo a pay period. Think about it-if you work a 40 hour work week and smoke a pack a day and you are able to stop smoking you will be giving yourself the equivalent of a 94 cent raise! That is almost a dollar raise! I have worked some places that take you 4 to 5 years or more to get a raise equal to that. $1825 a year could very easily help make a better vacation, upgrade to hd satellite tv, better clothes, whatever you do with that is money right now that is going to support killing you that could be going for a million other different things to better your life or the lives of your family.

I would dare say your toughest challenge in stopping smoking will be the social aspect and interaction with other smokers. There is a certain kind of camaraderie that goes along with smoking with others, a sense of belonging and of acceptance of that particular group you are with. You must remember that although it will be very difficult to hang around others smokers and be trying to quit. It can be done, I did it and if I can do it anybody can including you. If your friends are true friends they will accept your decision to stop smoking and pressure you or tempt you to try and fail. If you find your strength waning you may need to be absent from those friends and places on the temporary occasions when you feel extra weak. The other thing you will find difficult it that it may be a long time before you actually don't crave cigarettes. I think it was about a year for me before I didn't take a deep breath and remember how that cigarette was and how great it felt when the nicotine takes its effect through my body so instantly whenever I would see or be around someone who was lighting one or smoking one. At some point you have to decide is the pleasure of smoking worth more to you than better health.

Chapter Two

Seven Year Old Smoker

Yes, I know it is hard to believe but I personally started smoking at the ripe old age of seven! I know that is incredibly young and I don't what made decide to start doing it. You know how kids are about idolizing their parents and I had a Dad who smoked around 2 packs a day and I of course wanted to be just like him. I can remember when my Mom and Dad went to take a "nap" he would often leave his cigarettes on the table or the TV and I got the bright idea of sneaking one,

just one out of his pack. I figured he
would not miss just one. I would take
that cigarette and hide it under my bed in
a plastic colored baby bottle that was
under there. I would do this for several
days and when I had quite a few of them
I would plan my getaway to go play at a
friend's house but really go somewhere
else where I knew a teenage boy who
smoked and we would have a grand old
time! Man I thought I was really
something smoking and puffing on that
cigarette. I can remember being other
places and pulling my big old cigarette
and start smoking away on it and on
more that one occasion and adult or
someone older would say "That
cigarette's bigger than you are ain't it!" I
would just smile and puff away. I thought
I was big stuff and I liked the attention! I
will never ever forget what my body told
me that first day I actually inhaled. My
big "cool" teenage buddy observed me
smoking one day and said "You're not
inhaling that are you?" I said yeah and I
didn't know what he meant and he said

when you draw it into your mouth hold it in there and take a deep breath......OOHHHH My God in Heaven I thought I was going to die, choking and coughing and that rush of wooziness, pleasure and a sick feeling all mixed into one. You would think we would all have gotten a clue after that but no, we all went right on with it, glad to be in the club-the idiot's club!

I went on stealing cigarettes from my Dad when I could and I even sneaked a pack or two whenever he would buy and bring home a carton. I would always hit up people I knew who smoked for cigarettes as well and you how it is, most were happy to share back then. Yes I hate to admit but I have even went through the public ash tray and smoked my share of the leftover butts of others! Isn't it amazing what drug addiction will reduce you to?

I continued my smoking career of a pack a day all through high school and it wasn't until I got into college that I learned what all was actually in a cigarette! It is unbelievable what they contain. Everyone knows that smoking can cause cancer but when you really look at what is in them it is truly amazing that not every single person that smokes them doesn't get cancer. It shows just how remarkable our bodies are at fighting off the chemical and poisons we put in them.

A cigarette has over 3000 different chemicals and none of them are good for you. It has arsenic-rat poison, ammonia-toxic household cleaner, butane-from lighter, butyl acetate-a lacquer and enamel solvent, carbon monoxide, poison in car emissions, formaldehyde-embalming preservative for burial, methane-poisonous gas also used in rocket fuel, nicotine -the poison we all love. Now that think about all that the next time you fire one up!

If all the chemicals and carcinogens that

are in a cigarette don't solidify in your mind it is time to quit then you are probable not truly ready to lay them down just yet and if not that's OK. We have the right as free moral agents to make whatever choices we decide no matter how bad those choices are. The fact that you bought this book shows some positive and right thinking in the right direction that you are wanting to quit. The desire to quit once it gets strong enough will carry you through to do it at some point. Just be careful not to sabotage yourself with your mouth by being negative and thinking negative thoughts. If you don't first believe that you can quit you have already defeated yourself. If you go around saying I can't quit or telling yourself in your mind that you will never be able to quit, remember that is a lie you are telling yourself and whenever that thought comes into your mind or out your mouth stop immediately and think or say no, that's not right if I really have the desire to quit I can do it. Remember the millions that have gone before you and have been able to quit. I never had a problem quitting, for me it was staying "quit" that was the problem. I can remember throwing a half full pack away several times only to end up bumming and or buying a pack the very next day! One last thing you must and I mean you absolutely must must must do once you have been off of them for awhile and that is never and I mean never ever never ever take that first draw ever again. Every time I ever got back on cigarettes it was with just one draw off of someone's cigarette then the draw brought the thought just one cigarette won't hurt and BOOM you right back to square one and smoking again. I can not express to you strongly enough how vitally important it will be for you to never take that first draw once you are off of them. You must mentally prepare there will be bad days, stressful days, bad things that may happen, any number of circumstances may come up at any given time that are going to make you want to reach for a cigarette. DON'T DO IT!!!

Find any of a million other things to cope
with the situation besides lighting up a
cigarette because once you do give in
you will then immediately have the
frustration of having given in and so your
bad situation will only be compounded
by your giving into smoking again and
it's not worth to start all over again trying
to quit. Believe me I know the more time
you fail and give in the harder it is that
next time to not give in again.

Chapter Four

The Last Straw

I think the last straw for me to truly and finally make up my mind and set my mind to stop and stay stopped for good was when my body starting sending me the warning signals. I started having shortness of breath all the time. The lease little bit of exertion and I would be exhausted and out of breath. Then there was the hacking and coughing and the occasional phlegm ball that would come up. This really starting getting my attention and I started thinking you know I am really starting to not enjoy smoking anymore. I started worrying about cancer and how it would devastate my family and what a horrible way to die that would be. I had seen the smokers with late stages of emphysema   lugging around their oxygen tanks and still smoking! Unbelievable! I guess they figure once you have got that or lung cancer it is too late to quit and they are right. You might as well light em up baby! Once you get cancer or emphysema your chances are slim to none of recovering. Yes there are those who have their cancer go into remission but   for the vast majority it is their death sentence. When my brother got cancer I had all these high hopes that God was going to heal him. I am a very strong believer and I believe I have a very strong faith and I thought I just knew God was going to heal him and use him to travel around and tell his story of how God healed him. Well it didn't happen! God's way of healing him was taking him home to be with Him. I was so angry at God for not seeing things my way and please don't be offended, if you don't believe in God or a higher power I totally respect that. We are free moral agents and can believe whatever we want to in this life and we can agree to disagree and go on in love   and not worry about it.

Chapter 5

Are You Ready To Quit The Easy Way?

Well here it is, the easy way that I quit smoking. It really is a very simple way to do it and it worked for me and I hope and pray that it will work for you. I never was one of those people that could just lay them down and not pick them up again. If you can do that then that is great and congratulations but if you are like me and never could quit that way do not be discouraged there is hope for you yet and that is the way that I did it!

I was basically smoking a pack to a pack and a half a day and what I got to thinking about is that my body is now hooked on x amount of this drug nicotine and I did not start out from the beginning smoking that many. I was only smoking a few cigarettes a day and over the next few years got myself up to smoking a pack and a half a day so my theory was that if I slowly and gradually increased my addiction to nicotine I should be able to slowly and gradually reduce my addiction to nicotine and that is exactly what I did! I personally took a whole year to get off of cigarettes and you don't have to do it that if you think you do this plan faster it totally up to you.

What I did was started leaving half a pack of cigarettes plus one more out of the pack and putting them on my dresser in a plastic bag to keep them fresh. I did this about two months and then when I didn't miss the cigarettes I wasn't smoking I knew it was time to cut down a little more. For example track yourself and see just how many cigarettes you smoke a day. Is it 25, 30 or 50? It doesn't matter, what matters is getting that number figured out and reducing only by one. When you don't miss that one reduce by two then three then half a pack and so on. Remember that the slower you do this your body will not even notice the reduction because it will so slow and gradual.

I did this about every month to 2 months and after about 10 months I got down to smoking 3 cigarettes a day. Man those were the best cigarettes I ever smoked but I really wanted to quit so I continued downward until I got down to one cigarette a day and then when I was only smoking one a day I knew I had it beat. I smoked that one cigarette a day for about a month and a half and finally stopped and I kept a pack in my car and everything because you have to be able to be around and say no to them because you are going to run into every time you turn around. I know this is very simplistic but to therein lies its power. No money on pills with terrible side effects. No outrageous cost of nicotine gum etc. I just kept doing what I was doing over about a year's time and I have never smoked again since!

Remember you can do it! Just take the easy way, the sure and slow way and you will off of them before you know it!

I hope and pray this book
has been a blessing to you
and if you would like to
contact me I can be reached
at
art.guess@embarqmail.com

About the author

Arthur Guess resides in East TN with his wonderful wife of 17 years and 3 beautiful and wonderful children.